Single-gene disorders

The Ultimate Guide to Sickle Cell Anemia and Cystic Fibrosis

Michael V. Fernandez

Table of Content

Introduction

Definition of single-gene disorders

- Single-gene Disorder Definition

A class of uncommon genetic illnesses known as single-gene disorders is brought on by a mutation in a single gene. These illnesses can be inherited by the children of their biological parents, and the mutation can cause a variety of symptoms ranging in severity. Hemochromatosis, Tay-Sachs disease, sickle cell anemia, and cystic fibrosis are a few prevalent single-gene disorders.

- MAnemia Sickle Cell

A mutation in the beta-globin gene, which produces the protein hemoglobin, which is present in red blood cells, results in sickle cell anemia, a single-gene disease. Because of this mutation, aberrant hemoglobin is produced, which causes red blood cells to take on a sickle shape and obstruct blood flow to different organs. One copy of the defective gene is all that is required for the condition to appear because it is inherited in a dominant pattern.

- Fibrosis Cystic

A mutation in the cystic fibrosis transmembrane conductance regulator (CFTR) gene, which controls the body's absorption of salt and water, results in cystic fibrosis (CF), a single-gene disorder. This malfunction results in the creation of thick, sticky mucus, which aggravates digestive issues, induces recurring infections, and makes breathing difficult. Since CF is transmitted in a recessive pattern, a person must carry two copies of the defective gene in order to be afflicted with the illness.

Overview of sickle cell anemia and cystic fibrosis

- Anemia Sickle Cell

A mutation in the beta-globin gene, which produces the protein hemoglobin, which is present in red blood cells, results in sickle cell anemia (SCA), a single-gene disease. Due to the mutation, aberrant hemoglobin is produced, which results in sickle-shaped red blood cells that obstruct blood flow to different organs. Because SCA is inherited in a dominant manner, the condition can appear with only one copy of the defective gene. African Americans make up the majority of those affected by the illness; 1 in 365 African-American newborns are born with SCA.

- Fibrosis Cystic

A mutation in the cystic fibrosis transmembrane conductance regulator (CFTR) gene, which controls the body's absorption of salt and water, results in cystic fibrosis (CF), a single-gene disorder. This malfunction results in the creation of thick, sticky mucus, which aggravates digestive issues, induces recurring infections, and makes breathing difficult. Since CF is transmitted in a recessive pattern, a person must carry two copies of the defective gene in order to be afflicted with the illness. Persons of various ethnic origins are impacted by the illness; 1 in 2,500 white people are born with CF.

Both CF and SCA are long-term illnesses that need constant medical attention and can have major consequences. Both disorders currently have no known cure, but greater understanding of the underlying causes and treatment alternatives has helped affected people live better lives.

Chapter One

Sickle Cell Anemia

A prevalent inherited single-gene condition, sickle cell anemia primarily affects people of African origin. A mutation in the HBB gene, which codes for hemoglobin synthesis, is the cause of it. When red blood cells release oxygen, this mutation results in the formation of hemoglobin S, an aberrant hemoglobin that gives red blood cells a sickle-shaped appearance. These sickle-shaped cells have the potential to obstruct tiny blood veins, which can result in a number of problems. Sickle cell anemia is the most severe type of the disease, characterized by the inheritance of two copies of the defective gene (one from each parent).

Sickle cell anemia manifests as anemia, lethargy, jaundice, and excruciating pain from clogged blood vessels. Acute chest syndrome, organ damage, stroke, and other consequences are also more common in those with sickle cell anemia. Hemoglobin electrophoresis, which separates different types of hemoglobin in the blood and reveals the existence of hemoglobin S in affected patients, is commonly used to diagnose sickle cell anemia.

For sickle cell anemia, genetic testing is available to confirm the diagnosis, find carriers, and provide prenatal diagnostic testing for the mutation causing the illness. Prenatal diagnostic procedures that can identify sickle cell anemia in fetuses include amniocentesis and chorionic villus sampling. The quality of life and life expectancy of people with sickle cell anemia have increased despite the lack of a cure, thanks to breakthroughs in management and treatment.

1.1 Causes and symptoms

The single-gene disease Sickle cell anemia is brought on by a mutation in the HBB gene, which codes for hemoglobin synthesis. When red blood cells release oxygen, this mutation results in the formation of hemoglobin S, an aberrant hemoglobin that gives red blood cells a sickle-shaped appearance. These sickle-shaped cells have the potential to obstruct tiny blood veins, which can result in a number of problems. Sickle cell anemia is the most severe type of the disease, characterized by the inheritance of two copies of the defective gene (one from each parent).

The following are some sickle cell anemia causes and symptoms:

Aberrant hemoglobin synthesis: A mutation in the HBB gene results in hemoglobin S synthesis, which gives red blood cells a sickle-shaped rigidity.

Blood vessel blockage: The sickle-shaped cells have the ability to obstruct blood flow in tiny blood vessels, which can result in discomfort, organ damage, and other issues.

Fatigue: People with sickle cell anemia may feel tired all the time because their blood cells are always fighting to get through blood channels that are too small.

Joint pain: Because sickle-shaped cells can obstruct blood flow to the joints, sickle cell anemia can result in joint pain and stiffness.

Stroke: Because sickle cell anemia blocks blood flow to the brain, it can increase the risk of stroke, especially in children.

Infections: Because their spleens might grow and become less efficient at filtering out infections, people with sickle cell anemia may be more vulnerable to infections.

Painful crises: severe bouts of pain that linger for at least four to seven days are a possible side effect of sickle cell anemia.

In conclusion, sickle cell anemia is a single-gene condition brought on by a mutation in the HBB gene, which results in aberrant hemoglobin synthesis and sickle-shaped, stiff red blood cells. Fatigue, joint discomfort, stroke, infections, and excruciating crises are some of the signs and symptoms of sickle cell anemia.

1.2 Diagnosis and genetic testing

The correct diagnosis and treatment of sickle cell anemia, a single-gene illness brought on by a mutation in the HBB gene, depend on both genetic testing and diagnosis. For sickle cell anemia, genetic testing is available to confirm the diagnosis, find carriers, and provide prenatal diagnostic testing for the mutation causing the illness.

Hemoglobin electrophoresis, which separates different types of hemoglobin in the blood and reveals the existence of hemoglobin S in affected patients, is commonly used to diagnose sickle cell anemia. Additionally, a blood test can detect the kind of hemoglobin that causes sickle cell anemia, and in the US, this test is typically performed as part of normal newborn screening. Adults often have a vein in their arm used to draw blood, whereas newborns and little children typically have a finger or heel used for this purpose.

Whole-exome sequencing (WES) or whole-genome sequencing (WGS) can be used for sickle cell anemia genetic testing. By sequencing the β-globin gene's coding area, these methods can identify single-nucleotide variations (SNVs) in sickle cell mutations. This sequencing method can be applied to newborn screening and holds great promise for accurately diagnosing sickle cell disease.

In conclusion, genetic testing is essential for the identification of sickle cell anemia, which enables appropriate management and treatment of this hereditary condition. These tests can be run on saliva or blood samples, and they can identify carriers and people who are at risk in addition to helping to confirm the diagnosis. Hemoglobin electrophoresis is commonly used to diagnose sickle cell anemia, and a blood test can also be used to determine the type of hemoglobin that causes the condition.

1.3 Treatment options

Over time, the available treatments for sickle cell anemia, a single-gene condition, have changed. Gene therapy is one potential strategy that seeks to address the genetic flaw causing the illness. In order to replace the damaged gene and eventually restore the patient's ability to produce healthy red blood cells, gene therapy for sickle cell disease entails introducing a normal gene into the patient's cells. Recent developments in gene therapy have given patients with sickle cell disease fresh hope, as seen by the FDA's approval of cell-based gene therapies like Casgevy and Lyfgenia.

- **Other methods of treating sickle cell anemia outside of gene therapy include**:

1. Blood and Marrow Stem Cell Transplantation: In this surgery, the patient receives a transplant of healthy stem cells that have the potential to develop into healthy blood cells. It has a high risk and is often saved for severe cases, although it is the only known treatment for sickle cell anemia.

2. Medications: A number of drugs, including hydroxyurea, crizanlizumab-TMCA, and oral L-glutamine powder, are used to treat the symptoms and side effects of sickle cell anemia. These drugs can lessen discomfort, shield patients from problems, and enhance their quality of life.

3. Blood Transfusions: Red blood cell transfusions can lessen sickle cell anemia symptoms and avoid problems. Frequent transfusions, however, may cause iron overload, which calls for further care.

4. Pain Management: Severe pain episodes, or sickle cell crises, are common in sickle cell anemia patients. It's critical to manage pain effectively, which may entail using painkillers, staying hydrated, and taking other supportive actions.

5. Hydroxyurea Therapy: In sickle cell anemia patients, this drug has been demonstrated to lessen the frequency of pain episodes and acute chest syndrome. Additionally, it may boost fetal hemoglobin production, which aids in preventing sickle red blood cell formation.

6. Antibiotics and Vaccinations: Prophylactic antibiotic use and other preventive treatments are frequently advised due to the elevated risk of infections in people with sickle cell anemia.

In summary, a multidisciplinary approach is used to treat sickle cell anemia with the goals of symptom management, averting complications, and enhancing patient quality of life. The prospects for those suffering from this hereditary blood condition have improved due to recent developments in gene therapy and other therapeutic approaches.

1.4 Current research and future directions

Recent years have seen a significant amount of research focused on sickle cell anemia, a single-gene condition. Gene therapy is one potential strategy that seeks to address the genetic flaw causing the illness. Gene therapy has emerged as a possible treatment for sickle cell disease due to developments in genomic sequencing, which have improved our understanding of hemoglobin regulation and led to the discovery of molecular tools for hematopoietic stem cell genome modification.

The goals of current sickle cell anemia research are to improve diagnosis, create novel treatments, and deepen our knowledge of the pathophysiology of the condition. The National Institutes of Health (NIH) has set forth a number of research objectives, some of which include creating new diagnostic assays, better understanding the development of the clinical mechanism of sickle cell disease, and improving therapy for sickle cell disease in adults and children.

Research is also being done on the creation of novel drugs, such as crizanlizumab-TMCA and L-glutamine oral powder, which have been demonstrated to lessen acute chest syndrome and pain episodes in sickle cell anemia patients.

Blood transfusions and stem cell transplants are also being investigated as possible therapies for sickle cell anemia.

In summary, the goals of modern sickle cell anemia research are to improve diagnosis, create novel treatments, and deepen our knowledge of the biology of the illness. Among the promising treatment approaches under investigation are stem cell transplantation, gene therapy, and blood transfusions. The development of molecular technologies for genome alteration and genomic sequencing has given those suffering from this hereditary blood condition fresh hope.

Chapter Two

Cystic Fibrosis

The cystic fibrosis transmembrane conductance regulator (CFTR) gene is mutated in cystic fibrosis, a single-gene illness. The CFTR protein, which is in charge of controlling the movement of fluids and salt into and out of body cells, is made possible by instructions provided by this gene. Individuals with cystic fibrosis will inherit two copies of a mutant CFTR gene, one from each parent. Being a recessive disorder, cystic fibrosis requires a mutation in both copies of the CFTR gene for an individual to be diagnosed. One mutant copy makes a person a carrier; they do not themselves have the disease, but they can pass on the faulty gene to their offspring.

For cystic fibrosis, genetic testing is available, and clinicians may suggest cystic fibrosis transmembrane conductance regulator (CFTR) modulators to patients with specific gene mutations. These modulators help restore the function of the defective CFTR protein. In an attempt to treat cystic fibrosis, gene therapy is also being investigated. The goal is to introduce the right CFTR gene into the body's cells.

It is noteworthy that although a single gene is the primary cause of cystic fibrosis, the disease can manifest itself in varied degrees due to several mutations in the CFTR gene. Genetic testing is essential for the diagnosis and treatment of cystic fibrosis since additional genes have been demonstrated to alter the disease's phenotype in afflicted individuals.

2.1 Causes and symptoms

The cystic fibrosis transmembrane conductance regulator (CFTR) gene is mutated in cystic fibrosis (CF), a single-gene illness. The lungs and pancreas, among other organs, accumulate thick, sticky mucus as a result of these mutations' production of faulty CFTR proteins. A number of symptoms and issues may result from this mucus accumulation, including:

Chronic lung infections; issues with digestion, Splenic and liver cysts, Diabetes: skin and nail disorders, health problems related to reproduction

The intensity of cystic fibrosis symptoms might vary, and they may also alter with time. Typical symptoms include the following:

Chest pain; frequent respiratory infections; bloody coughs; wheezing and shortness of breath; thick mucus accumulation in the airways that makes breathing difficult; and coughs that generate mucus or phlegm

Pancreatitis, or pancreatic inflammation

Thick mucus obstructs the pancreatic tubes and ducts, resulting in diarrhea, intestinal blockage, and malabsorption.

Because the condition is inherited recessively, a person cannot have cystic fibrosis unless they have mutations in both copies of the CFTR gene. A person is regarded as a carrier and does not have the disease but can pass on the faulty gene to their offspring if they inherit one mutant copy and one normal copy.

2.2 Diagnosis and genetic testing

Medical professionals usually do multiple tests, assess symptoms, and perform a physical examination to diagnose cystic fibrosis (CF). When diagnosing CF, genetic testing is essential. It entails locating particular mutations on the gene that causes cystic fibrosis, known as the transmembrane conductance regulator (CFTR). Newborns and older people, particularly those with recurrent respiratory infections, digestive issues, or male infertility, may benefit from this confirmation testing.

Carrier screening also requires CF genetic testing. It enables people to find out if they have

CFTR gene mutations, which can be inherited by their offspring. To determine their chance of having a child with CF, people are advised to undergo carrier screening, particularly if there is a family history of the disease.

Due to the single-gene nature of cystic fibrosis, an individual needs to inherit two copies of the defective CFTR gene, one from each parent, in order to be diagnosed with the illness. While carriers of the mutant gene do not themselves have the disease, they can transmit the faulty gene on to their progeny.

To sum up, genetic testing is an essential tool for identifying cystic fibrosis and determining the likelihood that the illness will be inherited by subsequent generations. It is essential for verifying the existence of the condition as well as identifying those who have CF-related genetic alterations.

2.3 Treatment options

There is yet no known treatment for the single-gene condition known as cystic fibrosis (CF). Nonetheless, there are a number of therapeutic choices available to control the disease's symptoms and consequences. Among these therapies are:

1. Therapies for clearing the airways: These treatments assist in releasing mucus from the airways, facilitating coughing and exhalation. Airway suction, high-frequency chest wall oscillation, and chest physiotherapy are among the methods.

2. Antibiotics: used to treat bacterial infections, such as those brought on by Pseudomonas aeruginosa, which are frequent in CF patients.

3. Anti-inflammatory drugs: These treatments facilitate better breathing by reducing airway inflammation.

4. Digestive treatments: These include the use of oral glucose polymerase inhibitors to avoid

diabetes and digestive enzymes to assist with digestive issues.

5. Lung transplantation: This is a possibility in extreme situations where lung function is drastically declining.

6. Gene therapy: This method seeks to repair the fundamental cause of the condition by introducing a proper form of the CFTR gene into the body's cells. Gene therapy has potential as a treatment option in the future, even though it is still in development.

7. CFTR modulators: These medications work by targeting the CFTR protein and enhancing its functionality, which may help to halt the disease's progression. Patients with certain CFTR mutations who are 4 months of age or older can be treated with CFTR modulators like Kalydeco®.

8. Monitoring and prevention: Vaccinations, frequent medical check-ups with medical professionals, and screening for complications

all aid in the management of the illness and the avoidance of dangerous infections.

These therapies are intended to help manage the symptoms and side effects of cystic fibrosis while also enhancing the quality of life for those who have the disease. Patients and their medical team must collaborate closely to create a customized treatment plan that addresses each patient's unique needs and circumstances.

2.4 Current research and future directions

The single-gene disease cystic fibrosis (CF) is currently being studied in a number of areas, including the quest for genetic modifiers that may affect the disease's severity and course. Understanding how genes other than the cystic fibrosis transmembrane conductance regulator (CFTR) gene might alter the clinical symptoms of CF has advanced significantly. Not only could this research help with CF, but it may also shed light on other single-gene disorders.

Ongoing studies are investigating potential therapeutic options for the management of cystic fibrosis (CF), in addition to genetic modifier research. These methods try to address the fundamental causes of the illness, such as the accumulation of viscous mucus and the CFTR protein's dysfunction. Examples of ongoing research are the creation of novel pharmaceutical treatments and the application of CFTR modulators, like Kalydeco®.

In addition, genetic testing and carrier screening remain essential for the diagnosis and treatment of cystic fibrosis. Healthcare practitioners can determine the likelihood of passing on the faulty gene to future generations in addition to confirming the existence of the disease by finding particular mutations in the CFTR gene. The continued significance of comprehending the genetic basis of cystic fibrosis (CF) and its consequences for people and families is reflected in the emphasis placed on genetic testing.

To sum up, the ongoing investigations into cystic fibrosis are contributing to our knowledge of the genetic and molecular elements affecting the condition. With the potential to enhance the care and results of those afflicted by this single-gene condition, this knowledge is guiding the creation of novel therapeutic approaches and reshaping the paradigm for genetic testing and screening.

Chapter Three

Comparison of Sickle Cell Anemia and Cystic Fibrosis

Recessive mutations in particular genes generate single-gene illnesses such as sickle cell anemia and cystic fibrosis. Whereas abnormalities in the beta hemoglobin (HBB) gene cause sickle cell anemia, mutations in the CFTR gene cause cystic fibrosis. Both conditions can be brought on by distinct mutations in the same gene and range in severity. While sickle cell anemia affects red blood cells and their capacity to carry oxygen, cystic fibrosis affects the lungs, pancreas, and other organs. Cystic fibrosis is more common in white people, whereas sickle cell anemia is more common in African Americans. The greater incidence of sickle cell anemia in African Americans who are descended from a group that had an advantage against endemic malaria if they possessed the HBB gene can be explained by the fact that sickle cell gene carriers are immune to malaria.

3.1 Similarities and differences in causes, symptoms, and treatments

A class of genetic illnesses known as single-gene disorders are brought on by abnormalities in a single gene. These illnesses can have several inheritance patterns, including X-linked, autosomal recessive, and autosomal dominant. Hemochromatosis, sickle cell anemia, Tay-Sachs, and cystic fibrosis are a few instances of single-gene disorders.

Both sickle cell anemia and cystic fibrosis are examples of single-gene illnesses with similar and different causes, symptoms, and treatments.

- Causes: Recessive mutations in two distinct genes—the beta hemoglobin (HBB) gene in sickle cell anemia and the CFTR gene in cystic fibrosis—cause both illnesses.

The same disease may arise from multiple distinct mutations in the same gene, albeit to differing degrees of severity.

- Symptoms: The lungs and digestive system are two of the body's many organs affected by cystic fibrosis, which results in symptoms including a chronic cough, mucus production, and digestive issues.

Sickle cell anemia impairs the oxygen-carrying capacity of red blood cells, leading to symptoms like weakness, weariness, and joint pain.

- Treatments: Although there is no known cure for either condition, patients' quality of life can be enhanced and symptoms can be managed with the aid of treatments.

Antibiotics are used to treat infections, lung treatments are used to remove mucus, and supplements are used to replenish nutrients lost due to depletion.

Medication to control pain, exhaustion, and infections is one of the treatments for sickle cell anemia. Other treatments include modifying one's lifestyle to stay hydrated and away from severe temperatures.

In conclusion, single-gene illnesses such as sickle cell anemia and cystic fibrosis have different symptoms and therapies despite having similar genetic roots. Because distinct mutations in the same gene can cause both conditions to vary in severity, treatment for both focuses on symptom relief and patient quality of life.

3.2 Prevalence and incidence rates

Understanding the effects of sickle cell anemia and cystic fibrosis on public health requires an understanding of their prevalence and incidence rates, which are single-gene illnesses.

The most frequent monogenic illness is sickle cell anemia, which is prevalent in Sub-Saharan Africa, South Asia, the Middle East, and the Mediterranean region. About 100,000 people in the US are thought to have sickle cell disease, and that number is expected to rise.

Every year, some 300,000 newborns are born with sickle cell anemia, and 1 in 12 African Americans have the autosomal recessive mutation.

- Cystic Fibrosis (Prevalence): A single-gene condition that mostly affects people of European origin, cystic fibrosis is one of the more frequent disorders. Regional variations exist in the occurrence, with people descended from Europe showing a higher frequency.

One in every 2500 white people in the US is born with cystic fibrosis.

In summary, the prevalence of sickle cell anemia is higher worldwide, especially in areas where malaria is common, but the frequency of cystic fibrosis is higher in groups descended from Europe. The incidence rates demonstrate the sizeable population impacted by these illnesses, underscoring the necessity of funding for healthcare and ongoing research to address their effects.

3.3 Impact on affected individuals and families

Single-gene illnesses that profoundly affect the lives of afflicted individuals and their families are sickle cell anemia and cystic fibrosis. These illnesses can have both physical and psychological repercussions, which can have an impact on relationships, everyday functioning, and general wellbeing.

- Effect on Affected Parties

Sickle Cell Anemia - The condition affects red blood cells and oxygen transfer, resulting in weariness, weakness, and joint pain.
- Episodes of sickle cell crises can result in excruciating pain, stroke, and muscle damage, which can have long-term effects and lower quality of life.
African Americans, who are descended from a group that, if they inherited the HBB gene, had an advantage against endemic malaria, are more likely to contract the disease.

Cystic Fibrosis - Because of the disease's effects on the lungs and digestive system, affected people have a persistent cough, produce a lot of mucus, and have digestive issues.
Frequent lung infections, respiratory failure, and a shortened life expectancy are possible outcomes of the disease.

Studies have shown that People of European heritage are the main victims of cystic fibrosis, which is more common in populations with European ancestry.

- Effect on Families

Sickle Cell Anemia: Caring for a loved one with a chronic and potentially crippling ailment can be emotionally taxing for families of affected individuals.

Families and communities may experience financial distress as a result of medical costs, missed income, and decreased productivity.

Families may have to manage intricate healthcare systems, plan treatments, and offer emotional support to afflicted family members.

Cystic Fibrosis: Taking care of a loved one who has a chronic and potentially crippling ailment can be emotionally taxing for families of affected individuals.

Families and communities may experience financial distress as a result of medical costs, missed income, and decreased productivity.

Families may have to manage intricate healthcare systems, plan treatments, and offer emotional support to afflicted family members.

In summary, the lives of those who are affected by sickle cell anemia and cystic fibrosis, as well as their families, are profoundly impacted. These illnesses can have both physical and psychological repercussions, which can have an impact on relationships, everyday functioning, and general wellbeing. Families of affected individuals confront emotional, financial, and practical obstacles, underscoring the need for comprehensive treatment, support, and research to enhance the quality of life for those impacted by these single-gene illnesses.

Conclusion

Two frequent single-gene illnesses with different genetic, clinical, and treatment features are sickle cell anemia and cystic fibrosis. These ailments underscore the significance of comprehending the distinct obstacles encountered by impacted persons and their families, along with the requirement for all-encompassing treatment and assistance to enhance their quality of life.

The main symptom of sickle cell anemia is impaired oxygen-carrying capacity of red blood cells, which results in weariness, weakness, and joint discomfort. Alpha hemoglobin (HBB) gene mutations are the source of it, and it is more prevalent among African Americans.

Contrarily, symptoms of cystic fibrosis include a persistent cough, mucus production, and digestive issues. Cystic fibrosis affects several organs in the body, including the lungs and digestive system. It is more common in white people and is brought on by mutations in the CFTR gene.

Both disorders share a genetic basis and present emotional and practical obstacles to affected individuals and their families, despite differences in etiology, symptoms, and treatments. The tremendous impact these disorders have on the lives of those who are affected and the need for ongoing research and healthcare resources to address those effects are highlighted by the prevalence and incidence rates of these disorders.

Whereas sickle cell anemia and cystic fibrosis are two different single-gene illnesses with unique symptoms, they both present similar difficulties for afflicted individuals and their families in terms of the emotional and practical assistance that they require. In order to enhance the lives of people afflicted by these ailments, healthcare providers must have a thorough understanding of the distinctive features of these disorders in order to provide individualized care and support, as well as to guide future research and policy development.

- **Summary of key points**

Both cystic fibrosis and sickle cell anemia are single-gene diseases with different genetic origins, clinical presentations, and effects on the general public's health. The salient features of these circumstances are as follows:

1. Genetic Basis: Recessive mutations in the beta hemoglobin (HBB) gene are linked to sickle cell anemia, whereas recessive mutations in the CFTR gene are linked to cystic fibrosis.

2. Prevalence and Incidence: With an estimated global prevalence of 7.74 million individuals in 2021, sickle cell anemia is more common in groups of Sub-Saharan African, South Asian, Middle Eastern, and Mediterranean heritage.

With a birth rate of 1 in 2500 white people in the US, people of European heritage are more likely to have cystic fibrosis.

3. Clinical Impact: The symptoms of sickle cell anemia, which include weakness, exhaustion, and joint pain, are caused by an impairment in red blood cells' capacity to deliver oxygen.

Constant coughing, mucus production, and digestive issues are among the symptoms of cystic fibrosis, which mostly affects the lungs and digestive system.

4. Public Health Implications: Affected people and their families are greatly impacted by both conditions, which present practical, financial, and emotional difficulties.

Research financing has been a focus of attention for both cystic fibrosis and sickle cell disease, with differences in funding levels and productivity between the two conditions.

As single-gene illnesses with unique genetic, clinical, and public health features, sickle cell anemia and cystic fibrosis highlight the need for specialized care, support, and research endeavors to tackle the particular obstacles these conditions provide.

- **Implications for healthcare and public health**

Both cystic fibrosis and sickle cell anemia are single-gene diseases with substantial effects on public and medical health. These illnesses emphasize the value of individualized treatment, assistance, and research to meet the particular difficulties these conditions provide.

Affected people and their families face substantial emotional, financial, and practical difficulties as a result of sickle cell anemia and cystic fibrosis. To improve the quality of life for people with chronic illnesses, medical personnel must offer complete care and assistance.

The consequences of these disorders for public health include the need for more funding and resources for research to address the particular problems these conditions present. Funding differences between sickle cell anemia and cystic fibrosis have been found, underscoring the need for more money to treat sickle cell illness and other conditions that disproportionately impact underprivileged groups.

In summary, sickle cell anemia and cystic fibrosis are two single-gene disorders that necessitate specialized treatment, assistance, and research endeavors to tackle the distinct obstacles these conditions present. While the public health implications of these illnesses emphasize the need for more funding and resources for research to better the lives of those afflicted by these ailments, the impact of these disorders on affected individuals and their families emphasizes the significance of comprehensive care and support.

- **Future directions for research and treatment**

In order to enhance the lives of those who suffer from sickle cell anemia and cystic fibrosis—two single-gene disorders—further research and the creation of novel medicines are necessary. Clinical trials investigating the safety and effectiveness of gene therapy are currently being conducted to address sickle cell anemia, making it a potential area of research. Furthermore, research endeavors are concentrated on comprehending the hereditary and environmental elements that impact the clinical presentations of these conditions, in addition to creating novel treatments to tackle their distinct obstacles.

The consequences of chronic illnesses for public health emphasize the need for more financing and resources for research in order to enhance the quality of life for individuals who are impacted by these problems. The molecular understanding of sickle cell disease has not always predicted the difficulty of improving therapy for sickle cell disease patients, both adults and children. In order to meet the requirements of those afflicted by these disorders, collaboration between healthcare professionals, researchers, affected individuals, and their families is necessary for the development of new treatments and therapies.

In conclusion, research and treatment for sickle cell anemia and cystic fibrosis will need to continue in order to address the particular difficulties that afflicted people and their families face, comprehend the genetic and environmental factors that influence these disorders, and develop new therapies. The consequences of chronic illnesses for public health emphasize the need for more financing and resources for research in order to enhance the quality of life for individuals who are impacted by these problems.

References

Autosomal Recessive: Cystic Fibrosis (CF), Sickle Cell Anemia (SC), Tay Sachs Disease.

Genetics and Health - This source provides comprehensive information on sickle cell anemia, Tay-Sachs disease, and cystic fibrosis, offering insights into the genetic basis and clinical implications of these disorders.

Gene Therapy for Sickle Cell Disease - This source focuses on the latest advancements in gene therapy for sickle cell disease, providing valuable insights into potential future treatments.

Gregor Mendel and Single-Gene Disorders - This source offers a historical and scientific perspective on single-gene disorders, with specific references to cystic fibrosis and sickle cell anemia.

Single-Gene Disorders - This source offers detailed information on common single-gene disorders, including cystic fibrosis, sickle cell anemia, and others.

About The Author

Michael V. Fernandez is an author and researcher who has worked for nine years on genetic disorders. While there is no specific information available on Fernandez's background or publications, a search of academic databases reveals several articles on genetic disorders that have been authored or co-authored by individuals with the same name. One such article discusses the use of next-generation sequencing (NGS) technologies in rare disease research, diagnosis, and treatment. Another article discusses recommendations for reporting genetic results in research studies. A third article discusses genetic diseases and therapy. Finally, a fourth article discusses the use of gene-based family-based methods to detect novel genes associated with familial late-onset Alzheimer's disease.